Welcome to – **The Winning Mind Set For Weight Loss - The Thin book for Thin people**

This is a very practical weight loss guide to helping you lose weight; by the end of the book you will be able to have mastered control of your weight, understand your emotions and how to deal with them when they arise plus have a wonderful range of tools that you will be able to use on a regular basis to achieve successful weight loss easily.

Nearly all weight loss books say "run fast and eat lettuce". But we live in the real world where life and our inner voices get in the way of our being healthy all the time. What's inside this unique, practical and realistic weight loss book ?

- Learn easy mind exercises to take charge of your life.

- Find out the reasons why your weight goes up and down, and how to stop this easily.

- Discover the real secret of controlling weight and understanding your own language.

- Understand the implications of stuffing down and holding in your emotions and learn how to let them go

- Make your self-talk work for you in achieving weight loss success.

- Create a new slimmer and confident you, through the power of visualization.

Acknowledgements

To all the people that I have worked with that have achieved weight loss and gone on to a better and healthier lifestyle.

To the top athletes that I have coached who went on to win British and European Gold medals. It was a pleasure to work them and just shows that when you understand the sports science behind the how the mind and body work outstanding things can be achieved.

To the many clients I have worked with in using the Hypno-Band Gastric Band Surgery with the . This works very well because I examine the daily life of each client - look at what is not working, set goals, remove barriers, speak to the unconscious mind and agree new patterns that the client can then follow.

Thank you to all the clients and businesses I have worked with over the many years and continue to do so. I empower, encourage, motivate and inspire such lovely people to reach their goals in life. And at the same time I learn from each person I work with. There is no single way of working because everyone is special and unique.

Thank you to Marion McCrindle for all her help with this book.

Gary Sellors – January 2016

Index page –

I Think thin, Therefore I am .... Thin

Diet and nutrition experts emphasize that if you want to be healthier and have a trimmer, firmer body you should eat less and exercise more. We know that if you just burn more calories than you eat you will be successful. Your energy expenditure has to be greater than your intake. So, how do we start losing weight?

It all starts with your brain and what you are telling yourself. Your thoughts affect the way you think. The neuroscience side of you says that every negative thought you have is turned into a positive thought. An example: try NOT to think of a purple tree. You have to have had the thought of something to not think of something. Try it and see yourself.

This highlights the fact that thoughts create feelings and therefore control your behaviour. More scientists and health experts now accept this as we understand the mind and body more. The more we work with cognitive and behavioural therapeutic approaches the easier it is to achieve successful weight loss.

There are many different therapeutic interventions to help us lose weight and we will be discussing them throughout this book. They are easy to understand and learn and are very simple to use. We will start by examining those thoughts and negative behaviours that have held you back in the past.

It is said by psychologists that each of us thinks around sixty thousand thoughts as we go through our day. These thoughts are observing, analysing, creating, interpreting and remembering. It's amazing how complicated and distracting our thoughts can become. Do you remember a train of thought in your mind? Once the train starts off down the road of thinking negatively you find it very easy to add other carriages of the same type of thoughts.

These thoughts can at times be inaccurate or self-defeating. . Excellent mind tools like Neuro Linguistic Programming (NLP) can be of a great help to individuals to free themselves from the distortions and negative patterns that can shape peoples' lives.

If life was so simple that we could just sit on the sofa and think ourselves thin, losing weight (amongst other things) would be very easy. However, there is now a lot of scientific work around how the mind and body work. If we just combine a little action and increase our energy output, combined with the neuroscience side of thinking, we can get very positive results.

This book teaches you a new winning mind set for achieving success with weight loss. Using all of my therapeutic experience over 17 years and working with a range of clients and weight loss conditions. We will work on changing your thinking about what you eat and develop your understanding of the behaviours your thoughts create every day. It's an exciting time for you right now! Let's begin.

This book we will show you how to change your thoughts and change your feelings. We will encourage you through the tough times - and there will be some - but by working together and you doing the many different and yet very simple exercises in this book, you will achieve amazing results, look wonderful and lose weight.

What is Neuro Linguistic Programming (NLP) ?

NLP is a collection of a wide range of methods and models which create an understanding of thought process and behaviour. Understanding these techniques can bring about a positive change in you and others.

NLP stands for 'Neuro Linguistic Programming' and has been around since 1970's when its co-founders, Richard Bandler and John Grinder both modelled other therapists.

NLP is frequently known as the "users manual for your mind" and studying NLP gives us insights into how our thinking patterns can effect every aspect of our lives.

It looks at the way in which we think and process our thoughts (Neuro), the language patterns we use (Linguistic) and our behaviours (Programming) and how these interact to have a positive (or negative) effect on us as individuals.

The co-creators of NLP defined NLP as follows:

"NLP is an attitude which is an insatiable curiosity about human beings with a methodology that leaves behind it a trail of techniques." Richard Bandler (co-creator of NLP)

"The strategies, tools and techniques of NLP represent an opportunity unlike any other for the exploration of human functioning, or more precisely, that rare and valuable subset of human functioning known as genius." John Grinder (co-creator of NLP)

I have personally trained with Dr. John Grinder and Dr. Richard Bandler.

Which stage are you at ?

So where do you start? You start by taking one step at a time and always move forward. The important thing is maintaining your determination and being forward focused. There is much very interesting research over the last 15 years into how people change their habits and the effects of these changes. Behavioural scientists have for many years identified five stages that people go through when changing.

Originally proposed by Prochaska and Di Clemente in the field of smoking cessation, this model is commonly applied to thinking about weight loss, exercise, or other behaviours relevant to health.

It states that at any time, for any behaviour, individuals are at one of the following five stages of change behaviour:

Pre-contemplation - If you are at pre-contemplation stage you have not really thought about losing weight seriously, or literally have never thought about losing weight, perhaps because you think that you don't need to lose weight even though some of your friends may have mentioned it a few times. You have on the odd occasion found that you just cannot fit into some of your favourite clothes. They must have changed the sizes at the stores: you hear about it all the time. At this stage we are quite happy with our habits and lifestyle. Plus when we look around the town centre everyone seems to be the same size as you.

Contemplation – This stage is where you would really prefer not to lose weight, but slowly the reality is slowly creeping up on you. You have been to your local doctor and he/she has advised you to lose a little weight and exercise a bit more; perhaps your blood pressure has increased and you are huffing and puffing a bit more when you move a little quicker. Contemplation is about obstacles to change tending to surface their ugly heads. You notice that recent photos of you don't give you a good feeling about yourself; you look in the mirror on a rare occasion and suck your stomach in and say "I really should lose some weight". To change at this stage is about finding a motivational belief.

Determination – With liking the idea of losing weight, you are preparing yourself mentally - and often physically - for taking action to lose weight. You may have now joined a health club, approached a sports shop or at least asked advice from friends on the latest fitness clothing to wear. It wouldn't be surprising if a few health cook books have appeared on your book shelves. Also, you have decided to maybe to reduce the night time snacks. You have made a good decision here. Well done.

Action – You are moving forward, taking positive action and energetic steps to losing weight. Small changes in your lifestyle are beginning to show in a very positive way. You no longer take snacks to eat at your work desk; maybe you have started some calorie counting with the latest healthy app available on the market. You are on a mission and it's getting easier and not something that you are thinking about now. You are changing.

Maintenance - This is the magic, your continuing to go to the gym, even adding a few new classes. You are now strengthening, developing the positive results and changes that you have now successfully achieved. Whether or not you have reached your target weight, you have now made significant progress to losing weight.

Maintaining these behaviours can be at times very challenging, however, as we go through this book and look at a wide range of tools, you will be ready and prepared.

The four main key stages for losing weight

Pre-contemplation	Contemplation
1	**2**
Nothing's wrong with me. I don't need to do anything about my weight gain	I notice the clothes feeling a bit tighter, the photos of me don't make me feel great
Determination	**Maintenance**
3	**4**
I am taking a positive action towards losing weight, the new behaviours are starting to work.	All is going well and I am prepared for a fall back as I have a system in place to deal with this.

As you discover and know from past experiences and friends' tales, you will not go through this journey just once. Most people will go through the 4 main stages. Just like the circle of life, we are always learning.

However, as you go through this interesting book, learning a wide range of strategies to dealing with weight loss and how you can overcome the setbacks, you will become more aware and can plan for this. You will then find that these changes will become more permanent.

Preparation is the key. You will be ready and well prepared for success.

As you learn throughout this book, it's about the decisions you take and the choices you make. By the end of the book you are going to be in a wonderful position to be able to decide and make better decisions about losing weight, no matter what life throws at you. This book will help you achieve your goal of weight loss and ensure you have great strategies in place to support you in your weight loss journey.

Circle of weight loss excellence

NLP (Neuro linguistic programming) is an excellent exercise to use and can be adapted to many different areas of your life. Today we are going to use it effectively to help you lose weight.

You could also use this method to overcome fear of public speaking, to build up your confidence or if you want more motivation to exercise more or just need that mental lift. It really is a great tool. You will find it gives you the ability to sum up the confidence to use a skill you thought you didn't have.

Step 1. Stand in a nice space on your own and draw an imaginary circle on the ground in front of you, with you standing on the outside of it. Make the circle about 3 feet in diameter and 2 feet in front of you, the ideal size that you can stand in it. Some people like to actually draw the circle. You might use crystals or chalk - anything that makes it work for you. Once you know the shape and size of the circle you will be able to imagine it in your mind.

Step 2. As you stand outside the circle think about what's stopping you losing weight. Maybe it's a lack of money for gym fees, a lack of motivation or a lack of confidence to go to a local group for extra support/ join a running group. Find the major fear that's stopping you losing weight and as you do this pinch a finger and thumb.

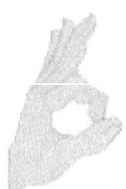

Really focus on this image of disappointment and keep pressing that finger and thumb. Then release. Press again to see if you still have that thought then release again. Well done.

Step 3. Now step inside the circle and imagine a time when you felt great about yourself or a time when you laughed so much your side hurt. Hear what you heard, see what you saw, feel what you felt. Take a big deep breath and say the word *NOW*. Step back out of the circle into your original position.

Step 4. As you stand there outside the circle of weight loss excellence, think of another issue that's stopping you losing weight. Be really honest with yourself. When we do this, we always know what the real reason is. Remember no one else knows what you are thinking. As you think of the barriers to your weight loss, press the same finger and thumb again and capture that REAL reason. Got it? You are doing amazing work; keep at it. Remember to release the fingers again.

Step 5. Now step back in the circle of weight loss excellence. Once again remember to think of another feel-good time. Your brain cannot tell the difference between imagination and reality, so all you have to do is make it up. Attach some emotion to it; brighten the image with wonderful colours and dream like a child would. Capture this feeling of emotional excellence using whatever role models or scenario work for you. Have fun with this. When you have it, take another deep breath and say the word *NOW*. You are doing great; almost there.

Step 6. Nowurn around in the circle of weight loss excellence. Look at your starting position outside the circle and how negative that position was. Here is the magic......... As you take a deep breath and say the word *NOW*, I want you to jump, Yes I did say jump.. out of the circle and back to the starting position. As you do this, press your finger and thumb together just like you did before. Keep them pressed and as you jump on the old spot now in the past, say the word *NOW* over and over again. As you jump up and down outside the circle you will feel AMAZING and those negative thoughts that have stopped you up until you did the exercise are now going into the past where they will remain.

Step 7. All is gone. Now step to a new position somewhere else outside the circle anywhere - it does not matter; the work is done. Look at the first position and notice how different you now feel. Then look inside the circle and relive those happy thoughts and feeling, and don't be surprised if you get drawn to jumping back in the circle, if so ... enjoy. It your new life..........

Repeat this exercise. whenever you feel the need to do; you will be amazed how easily it can be adapted.

Setting realistic and practical weight loss goals

The key here is setting you goals that are both realistic and practical. There is a lot of science that tell is that simply sitting on your sofa and wishing "I am thin, I am thin" doesn't work as well as taking some positive action. Let's look at what works well and show you how to set successful goals.

Setting goals is an important part of achieving effective weight loss. I always look at each client's case history and lifestyle and see what areas we can change quickly and what areas will need more time. It's important to have a very clear picture of how you will lose weight. It's important to know all the steps and have successful strategies in place for when you have a fall-back or when an emotional trigger is alerted.

I always recommend when planning a healthy weight loss programme that setting a realistic goal of 0.5kg per week is more than achievable. Everyone knows someone who has lost 7 pounds in a week on a diet - that latest fad diet and then when you see them months later they have gained more weight than when they started. The basic premise is - eat less and exercise more your energy output has always got to be greater than your energy intake. Let's help you keep it simple. This works.

It's so important not to think too far ahead. For example "I want to lose 3 stone in 6 months" etc.. This is a large amount of weight loss over a relatively long period but it has little meaning in respect of what you are going to do next. Let's keep it simple. You will achieve that 3 stone weight loss when you lose 0.5kg a week. I keep saying it LETS KEEP IT SIMPLE.

Little and effective steps constantly moving forward will keep you motivated, interested and passionate about your goals. Time will pass by quickly. Remember the neuroscience bit we discussed before. The brain does not understand negatives. If you keep saying "I must lose weight" your focus is on being overweight. If you say instead, "I am enjoying my new healthy regime" your focus is as it says. Change your mind set, change your body. Let's keep it simple.

Now you are in the achievable goal setting mind set let's see what else you can do. Focus your mind on other thoughts that will support your weight loss targets or your new healthy lifestyle. Remember you get more of what you focus on. Never forget this because it is key to achieving life's goals.

Let's look at why you want to lose weight. Understanding this is a vitally important element of the process because when the going gets tough, it is this aspect of your motivation that will help you through.

When I work with people who want to give up smoking, I ask them the same question. *Why do you want to give up smoking? W*hen their answer is,
"*my partner/husband/wife, wants me to give up*" because they don't smoke, what do you think their motivation is? When this happens with my clients, I stop the session. It's not going to work.

I kindly ask them to go away and re-think about giving up and only when they are ready and WANT to give up, should they come back. They always thank me for my honesty.

I could have taken their money, knowing it wasn't going to work but that is something that I not prepared to do. My work here in this book is realistic and practical for you losing weight.

So back to the WHY?

Is it because you want

- the energy to play with my children in the park
- to be able to fit in that nice dress in the window
- to be able to feel great and get noticed more
- to reduce the risk of having health problems later on in live

Or

- You have simply made a decision; your life is changing for the better.

That's a wow moment for many people. It can be the light bulb moment when you make these decisions. You just notice an amazing change in yourself. Don't be surprised if your breathing changes as you have that life-changing thought, because you have changed inside. This is very powerful work

Start by setting and frequently visualising your goals. See them, hear them, feel them and link them to your new positive healthy lifestyle and achieving your weight loss target.

I would recommend keeping a journal of your journey. This works very well because rather than having the thoughts going on in your mind, if you get them outside your head and put them down on to paper, you will find that you have more space in your brain to think healthier thoughts. It's always interesting if you list everything:

- What you eat
- What thoughts you had while you were eating
- How much you spend on food and drink
- Why you feel you should eat
- What your cravings are about

The other important thing is to highlight what's working well:

- Which exercise is working well?
- What have you noticed about your positive thinking?
- What supportive comments have you received this week?
- How more aware of your thinking are you?

Affirmations that will help you lose weight.

Most people are familiar with the quote by Emile Coue, ***"Every day, in every way, I am getting better and better."***

What people don't realize is that Emile Coue was a pharmacist and a pioneer in hypnotherapy. Emile believed in "autosuggestion" otherwise known as self-hypnosis. What he learnt through practice and time was that people responded better to remedies where they were supplemented by positive suggestions.

He was known to state that each person had within themselves the solution to their own problems. I truly believe this. The body knows how to heal itself. I have often said to clients that they already know what is stopping them losing weight; they just need to be honest with themselves.

Listed below are just a few "auto suggestions". Start to repeat them as often as possible - maybe write them down in the kitchen or carry them in your purse/wallet. After a while you will remember them without looking. If some affirmations just don't seem to work for you, that's fine; not all affirmations are for everyone. Each of us is unique. Enjoy.

Affirmations for Weight Loss

- I choose to exercise regularly every week
- I am the perfect weight for me
- I choose to make positive healthy choices for myself now

Affirmations for Love

- I rejoice in the love I encounter everyday
- I know that I deserve love and now I accept it
- I give out love and it is returned to me in multiple ways

Affirmations for Health

- Every cell in my body vibrates with energy and health
- Good health and wellness are mine now. I release my memories from the past
- Loving heals my life. I nourish my mind, body and soul
- My body heals quickly and easily

A good one I use is – *"The universe takes away all emotions, thoughts and feelings that I do not need for my body"*. (Louise hay)

Exercise more or eat less? - The chicken or the egg; which came first?

Some people would rather cut down on what they eat than work up a sweat at the gym or in the local park. Others prefer to exercise hard 5-6 times a week and not worry about what they eat. So which one works better? It really depends on what your goals are. Or can you do both?

There are no guaranteed recipes for good health although you will find that a combination of an interesting healthy eating plan coupled with a good dose of regular exercise are the ultimate recipe.

Everyone knows that regular exercise or physical exercise that involves movement such as gardening or walking helps the body function better and can help improve and reduce the risk of heart disease, diabetes and other unwanted health issues. It's good to be physically active on a daily basis because keeping active.

- helps protect you from developing heart disease and stroke or its precursors like high blood pressure

- improves the chances of living longer and living healthier

- can help the prevention of the insidious loss of bone density (known as osteoporosis)

- contributes to lifting depression and anxiety mood swings

- helps improve sleep

We all know the term "couch potato" although it is not just aimed at people who don't do any physical activity. There have been many studies linking watching television and obesity. Research which monitored the diet and activity habits of 50,000 middle aged women over a period of 6 years showed that for every 2 hours the women spent watching television each day, 23 percent had a higher risk of becoming obese and 14 percent had a risk of diabetes.

The research showed that it didn't matter how much exercise they did. If they watched a high amount of television (and were thus inactive) there was an increased risk of obesity and diabetes.

Cutting back on television and computer time and other sedentary pastimes is just as important as becoming more active.

Other research shows that a brisk walk between 15- 20 minutes a day starts to decrease the chances of your having a heart attack or stroke or developing diabetes. Remember, a simple walk at a decent pace - enough to increase your heart rate and make you breathe deeper - will have a huge benefit to your achieving weight loss.

A tip is do not think too much about planning at first; just get outside and walk. In no time at all you will be surprised how time flies. Something I like to do is carrying a small camera with me and become an amateur photographer. Notice when you are walking down the high street just how many people are looking at the ground.

The physiology of the eyes says that when you look down you are accessing negative and positive emotions and when you look up you access the visual cortex which provides the pictures in your mind. This is very simple to do and yet so effective and very powerful. So next time you are feeling down and in a negative state of mind, notice that you looking down and move your eyes upwards, then you will break the state change. It's nearly impossible to cry when you look up.

One way to determine what "moderate activity" actually is, is to take the "talk test". This is when you are exercising enough to break a sweat (or "perspire" for the ladies) but it's not so uncomfortable that you cannot have a conversation with the person exercising next to you.

You simply do not realise how much time has passed. So chat away; just make sure you are moving forward as you do. Keep the exercise simple – just walk!.

Walking is a good starting exercise for many people as it's free and doesn't require any equipment. You can do it at any time of the day and night and in any place as long as you are safe. And its fun!

If you want to avoid the "middle aged spread" that most people of a certain age fear, physical activity is important. So is watching what you eat. Remember what we discussed before. Your energy output has got to be greater than your energy intake. Many people may need more than 2 hours of moderate intensity activity a week to maintain their current weight.

Another thing to be aware of is when your body plateaus and disappointment starts to kick in. Don't allow yourself to get stuck in a rut with your exercise. As your body adapts to exercise and you get more comfortable, you will need to change your routine just slightly - I would say about every 6 weeks. You need to push yourself more and more to get the same cardiovascular workout.

Another way to know that you need to change things is if you see your weight or waist size increasing. Just simply do the routine a different way; add bits or take away exercises. Remember: the brain is learning all the time. Keep it busy and wondering what you are going to do next. This will keep it fresh and your will find variety makes the exercise more fun as well.

Exercise is one of those rare things where . ood regular exercise is arguably the best thing you can do for your health and is a major element in achieving your weight loss. Any amount of exercise is better than none. Try running; it's free. Just do 5 minutes at first. Start walking then break into a gentle jog and build up from there. You can do it.

"Goal Setting:

1 - Set Long Term Goals

2 - Set Short Term Goals

3 - Set Objectives

4 - Prioritize the Objectives

5 - Define and Detail

6 - Do It

7 - Evaluate

Anonymous

Dealing with your inner voice

When we want to achieve a successful weight loss we need to understand what we are telling ourselves. You know: _that_ inner voice - and yes, we all have one; you're not going mad! - that chatters to us all day long.

The words we hear ourselves say can be very negative although we don't mean to be negative. As we have discussed, the brain does not understand negatives. Everything we say to ourselves – for example…"_I will never lose weight", "exercise is hard work" or "I'm never going to get my shape back t_his self-talk just confirms to the brain that this is true. The brain makes it a positive and gives it back to you in bucket loads - hence why it's really important that you control your thoughts and inner talk.

Let's look at words that are no use to us which we say a lot. I'm sure you remember saying to yourself that you are "planning" to go to the gym or "planning" to go on a diet". Or a good favourite is "I'm trying" to get a better figure. Do these words ring any bells? And how many times do you say them every day to yourself? We find these words create doubt or can show ambivalence. You find yourself accepting what is happening. Let's remove these kinds of words from our inner talk and replace with more proactive talk, so as to enable you to lose weight more successfully. "I am losing weight" is a lot better than "I would _like_ to lose weight". Let's get you thinking more positive and see more active verbs such as _be_ and _do_ in your new language.

Once you realize the massive influence of the thoughts you have and the amazing new lifestyle you could have if you could control them, you will be in a stronger position to STOP living your old lifestyle with those old limitations in your language.

Change your thoughts, change your body. When you make this jump forward into a more positive approach with the right kind of language, your weight loss target will be reached and you will notice that your life will be filled with interesting opportunities, potential and fulfilment as a result of your taking more control and creating the reality you desire.

When you are thinking and talking about your weight loss struggles and what's not working, look at switching to the past tense. "I'm just too lazy to lose weight" change it too "I used to be too lazy to lose weight" or when you have told yourself "I am so unattractive because of my weight" this now becomes "I used to be so unattractive because of my weight". You are not the you of the past. Just remind yourself that you have changed; you are capable of new changes and now, in fact, you are already changing for the better and face a more positive future.

The positive inner self-talk that you have with yourself shows that you believe in yourself and can feel confident in your capabilities to the point where you can be certain that you will succeed with your weight loss. You need to start saying " I am changing the way I live my life" or " I am losing weight easily" or "I am more eating healthfully".

Now that you realize that your inner talk has been going on since you were born, it's important for you to regain control over that inner voice. This does not happen overnight. However, as we have discussed before, with your determination to regain control, you are now changing that voice and mind set.

Another area to look at is the "why" you eat more than you should or "why" you don't go down the gym or "why do I just keep eating when I know I should stop". Some of the answers that might come to mind are, "that you are bored" or "things aren't going well for you right now".

Another word to look at is "how? "How do I over eat?" which might you might receive an answer. Such as. "I always eat something when I watch television" or "I don't have the money to buy better foods, so I buy rubbish cheap food". I'm sure some of these sayings will ring alarm bells but at least you are now beginning to become aware of them.

By becoming an observer of your inner talk you are going to be better placed to assess its validity (or lack of) and be able to challenge your thinking patterns. Also, over time, you will be more adept in seeing common trends and daily triggers that cause the negative inner talk to start and be able to use your new abilities to regain control.

People who are struggling to achieve their desired weight loss often sabotage themselves by saying things like "if" or "if only". An example of this would be, "if I could just lose 20 pounds" or "if only I could get myself down the gym" As we have discussed before, these types of comments simply reinforce the barriers to your weight loss. They focus on the effort you need to make rather than encourage you to take the first steps. If you start saying "I am starting to lose 20 pounds" and "I am now enjoying working out", this simple and yet very effective switch sets the way forward for you to believe that you can change your lifestyle and lose the weight.

Another little tip I recommend for regaining control of the voices is that when you are listening to them chatter away and feel you are starting to take sides with the negative one because its arguments seem sound, say "STOP!" Tell the voices that you have heard everything that have said both negative and positive, and tell them, "Thank you for your comments and advice, however, I choose to make my own decisions". Now you are really taking control of your life. Well done you.

It gives you a sense of pride in your accomplishment and a great sense of control over your life. It's an incredible boost to your confidence.

We are very much creatures of habit. So it's no wonder how easily we fall into patterns of self-destructive inner talk which affects our thoughts and behaviours.

Instead of continuing to be your own worst critic learn to teach yourself to be the best support mentor for yourself. Be respectful to yourself and treat yourself with the same compassion and kindness that you would treat others around you. NEVER say anything with your inner voice that you wouldn't want another person to say to you.

Great weight loss exercises.

Here are two great weight loss exercises for you to do; both are very powerful.

The Mirror Exercise – for seeing the new slimmer you

Find a nice place where you can be alone and not be disturbed. You can do this exercise standing or sitting down. Now imagine a full length mirror in front of you. Look at the mirror and see yourself standing there. Ignore any negative inner voices as discussed in the other chapter. Let's continue.

In the mirror is the new you. Notice how you look, what you are wearing; notice the bright colours. Allow yourself to really imagine the new you. Remember what we have discussed previously. If you play it out in your mind your brain will think you have done it and therefore it will become real. Notice how you feel?. Notice how you are now standing more confident. Notice what you are thinking as you look at the new you.

When you have this image of just how you are going to look in the near future, I want you to step into the magic mirror and step into yourself, like putting on new suit. Notice how it feels, the new you - at the bright colours that you don't normally wear. Look out through the eyes of the new you who is now you: see all around you. Hear the great compliments you are getting from family and friends as they compliment you on your new figure; notice your feelings and thoughts and enjoy this wonderful sensation.

When you are really comfortable with the new you and how great you now look. Step out of this image in the mirror and return to the start again, still noticing the new image of you in the mirror. Thank the new you for allowing you to experience this powerful opportunity and know that you can step into the mirror any time you need a confidence boost. Now I want you to imagine a large pink heart surrounding the mirror, as if by magic.

See the pink heart around the mirror and the image of the new you floating off into the distance and disappearing far, far away.. .

This is a very powerful exercise: notice how differently you now feel about the changes in your life.

The Rubber Band Snap – Exercise

Wear a rubber band on your wrist, any colour will do, and each time you hear negative inner self-talk in your mind say "Stop"! If you can't say "Stop" out loud pull the rubber band and let it snap back on your wrist. Be repeating this action, it will quickly remind you not to stay in that negative mind set and allow you to move on. This is a very effective alternative. The snapping of the band on your wrist creates the physical pain you feel, this will become a huge motivator to stopping your negative self-talk.

Do both of these exercises as many times as you feel necessary, and remember to have plenty of fun doing them. Both will have a positive impact on your weight loss progression.

Coaching yourself

This is a really good little exercise to do now and then; you will be surprised by what you get up to. Imagine you went and watched yourself in a coaching session; the "coach" is also "you" and will monitor what you get up to and what you're thinking about your lifestyle and what you eat.

The coach (your alter ego) would notice what you get up to with your eating habits and those little secret munchies when you know no one is looking; maybe it's when you are preparing the family meal at lunchtime or in the evening. Do you have a little nibble on a cake, biscuits or crisps?

Maybe you rush your food without noticing it or eating watch television and not concentrating on the food in front of you. If there is a nice cake in the house, just sitting there, you can't just leave it alone until it's all gone. Your coach might notice that when you seem to have negative thoughts you reach for the emotional foods without thinking about it. It can be quite an eye opener when you monitor yourself. You maybe be shocked by the results the coach notices.

To maximise the benefits of self-coaching to build on what you learn to enhance your weight loss coach yourself over the next 7 days. Monitor your thoughts, feelings and more importantly your behaviour.

Draw up a diary for your coach to track the results. (see below)

	Thoughts	Feelings	Behaviour
Monday			

	Thoughts	Feelings	Behaviour
Tuesday			

	Thoughts	Feelings	Behaviour
Wednesday			

	Thoughts	Feelings	Behaviour
Thursday			

	Thoughts	Feelings	Behaviour
Friday			

	Thoughts	Feeling	Behaviour
Saturday			

	Thoughts	Feeling	Behaviour
S u n d a y			

Once you have a full diary of thoughts, feelings and emotions, this will give you an understanding of areas that can be addressed as we go through this book.

The key is that the more honest you are with yourself and the degree to which you become aware of what you eat and why you eat it, the more successful you can be in changing your eating habits.

Parts Therapy exercise for you to do.

This exercise is amazing.

- Find a space where you can relax, where you will not be disturbed. Put on some relaxing music, close your eyes and now begin to relax

- Imagine that your excess weight is sitting in a chair right in front of you. When that image forms in your mind notice what you see, what you hear, what you feel. What colour is it? Describe the shape, size and shape?

- If that your weight could talk, what would it say? If it is reluctant ask your unconscious mind, what do you think it would say?

  (by asking this question you are bypassing the conscious mind and dealing directly with the subconscious mind, the good stuff)

- If it could tell you about itself and the role it is playing in your life what would it say?

- Now pretend you are the weight. Be in the chair, be the weight and look straight ahead and see yourself............ (your name). What can you tell yourself about what role you play in your life so you can understand it better?

- Now be the real you… (your name) and respond to what the weight just said. Start a conversion between you and the weight.

- A good tip is when you get an answer, repeat the answer back and add "because"? as this will allow more information to come forward.

- When you repeat this with both parts, you realise that you both want the same thing.

- This is the middle ground allowing both parts to work together, without each part losing face.

- At the end of this exercise you will be in a position to understand what both parts are about, plus have a new agreement allowing you to go forward and work together.

- From my experience I have found this parts therapy exercise to be very interesting and powerful.

Meal planning

Let's now look at the way you plan your meals, for dinner, lunch and breakfast. It's been proven many times *"that a failure to plan is a plan to fail"*. This area can be one of the most important parts of losing weight and reaching your targets. We often know of people who plan a month in advance and cook a lot of food to freeze in little boxes.

That can be seen as good planning by some people and seen as boring by others. Both are right: it's whatever suits your life and work style. There is no best formula. The key thing is to have a strategy in place otherwise the chances are that you will fail. Then again, if you don't buy snacks, crisps and chocolates then you cannot eat them when bored or when a bit of negativity creeps in.

A lot people buy snacks on the way home. This means that they spend more money and buy more than they really need. Also – and more importantly - they are over eating. It is a known fact that you should never shop for food while you are hungry as you will always be tempted to buy more.

There is a 20 minute cycle that goes on in the thought processes of the brain. If you are hungry but don't react to the hunger pains / cravings you will be pleasantly surprised to find that you probably won't feel hungry anymore despite the fact that 20 minutes have passed and you haven't eaten anything. It works and is true.

Success to meal planning is following a process that you find enjoyable, one that is practical to your lifestyle and effective for you. More and more people are enjoying reading cook books or watching The Great British Bakeoff.

With today's technology and computers, tablets and available apps and the of food blogs available on-line there is a great easily accessible source and wealth of food planning advice. This can be very inspirational and exciting and at times can stimulate the brain into developing creative food ideas with which you can amaze your friends. Let yourself be inspired.

Do whatever works for you; don't fall into the trap of following everyone else. Never forget that we are all different and that fad diets and the latest quick fix rarely work in the long term, as we have discussed before. Your energy put has always got to be greater than your intake of food.

With the regularly changing weather that we have in the UK, adapt your food shopping to what's in season at the local market. Try new fruit and vegetables. Given that today a lot of food is grown in large green houses it's possible to get salad and healthy fresh food all year round. Don't forget the local market stall on the corner in the town centre; they have many great bargains and cheap, fresh foods to enjoy.

Also, if you have never asked for just 1 apple, 1 orange and/or 2 tomato before, you may be surprised to find that most markets stalls will gladly sell them to you. You don't have to buy a pound or kilo of everything.

As you build up your meal planning over, say, a year or at least 6 months, the records you have kept can become a good cook book to look back on later. You will be amazed by some of the things that you will have forgotten. Also, as you keep your food records and keep reviewing and editing meals that don't now fit in with your new healthy style, you will find that you have a wonderful very healthy personalized meal planning recipe book.

When planning your meals it can be fun to have a theme going through the week. Monday is salad, Tuesday is meat, Wednesday is fish etc. This will help you keep focused and in control when you have to make household changes and quick recipe decisions. When you go shopping, take the prepared shopping list and stick to it. You don't need all those other tempting foods. Remember: *YOU ARE NOW IN CONTROL.*

It can get overwhelming when you open the fridge door and stuff starts falling out. We tend to miss what is at the back, lost behind the pickles and sauces. Do not let things go bad. Aim to keep your fridge light and airy. Perhaps you might put a sticky note on the outside of the fridge to remind you of the food that needs to be eaten, because out of sight is out of mind. Simple and yet it's true for successful weight loss.

Meal planning is about being flexible, adaptable and having good back up strategies.

Have this in place and your weight loss and healthy lifestyle will be successful. Remember, "A failure to plan is a plan to fail".

"Listen closely: the only time it's too late to change yourself is when you're dead. Until then, you're simply making excuses or lying to yourself."

Anonymous

Are you in or out of control of your success with weight loss?

Are you really in control of your destiny and achieving a successful weight loss plan? Do you see yourself as the driver of your life going forward, or do you think that you cannot change what happens in your life? Never forget the neuroscience side of things that I have already mentioned. The brain cannot tell the difference between reality and imagination.

Which therefore brings us back to the key question - Are you in control or out of control? The choice is yours. A phrase I often say to my clients is *"You always have 2 choices. You can change things, or accept what you have, BUT... don't sit on the fence and moan about it".* Let's look at where your control is.

Internal thoughts and feelings

This is about you taking responsibility for your weight. You are saying things like "if I don't lose my weight, it's all my fault" or "the reason I have lost my weight is due to the exercise regime I have set myself". This shows that you are taking responsibility and thus your thoughts and actions have a direct influence on your actions. You are in a strong place of accountability and because of this you are able to correct your thoughts, feelings and behaviours. This is going to have a very positive impact on your weight loss plan.

However, if you are too focused inwards the downside - which can work against you sometimes - you can fall into the trap of not allowing outside resources to move you forward. Some people find it difficult to ask for help, listen to guidance from others or even gain knowledge from nutritionists and healthcare specialists.

Because of intense internal thinking, you can create your own problems and not find a way out of this; you tend to analyse your failures in respect of weight loss and, in some cases, you could make them bigger than they really are. It is possible, however, that you will not realise this as you believe your thinking and only your thinking is correct. This in turn will conceal your limitations and reduce your chances of success.

The key is to beware of this happening and work out how to change it.

When things happen beyond your control e.g. traffic problems, the weather or family changes, you need to be aware that you will be starting to think inappropriate thinking and you may, at times, start blaming yourself for changes that are well beyond your control.

Also, within the sphere of weight loss you need to be conscious of factors such as muscle changes due to your new exercise regimes or water retention. You may find that you have reached a plateau and you may have forgotten to change your exercise routines. I would recommend doing a different exercise routine every 6 weeks. This keeps it interesting and keeps your brain and body guessing what is going to happen next. Aim to be realistic about what is going on and how good you feel about your success.

Failure to acknowledge and accept your own actions and beliefs.

Some people cannot accept compliments and consider any success is due to external factors and not their own hard work. Similarly in life we have choices and we need to accept responsibility for those choices. These two elements can seriously get in the way of successful weight loss.

An example of the negative effect of modesty would be if your family or friends notice your regular weight loss and the fact that you are looking amazing. Because of external thinking you will say it's because of the latest diet which is on TV or in the magazines. In this thinking you haven't taken credit for your success.

It was all because of the diet and not your actions, or maybe because you have a great nutritionist, or have followed the advice your GP prescribed. This thought process shows that you take no ownership for the success with your weight loss.

An example of the second element – the failure to accept - would be if you put on weight and started to blame the calories in the foods that you eat saying that they have changed. It is nothing to do with your overeating on a regular basis or binge eating. It will always be linked with other people, situations and circumstances; therefore, you never own your thoughts and actions. No matter what the situation or circumstances, you just blame everyone else - even if the fault is purely your own doing.

If these ways of thinking continue you could be misunderstanding or avoiding the real reason why you are not losing weight. Unless you diagnose the correct reasons for not losing weight you will find that your coping strategies will also be wrong and hence ineffective.

This is why I have said before, it's important to remain in control.. It's important that you give yourself a reality check because until you do and accept that you are responsible for your decisions and actions you will struggle with losing weight. TAKE CONTROL NOW.

Your solution here is moving your focus of control from external to internal - from factors you feel you cannot control to factors you determine you WILL control. Once you start working on this area, the changes working towards your weight loss will be massive and very rewarding.

The problem with listening and watching external forces when looking for a perfect weight loss solution is that we are attracted to the latest diets or fads. But by doing this we are not taking control of our thoughts and bodies but entering a cycle which just goes up and down with no real result. This happens because there is no change to your thinking or behavior and hence, when the diet is "finished", there is a high chance you will revert to your former patterns of thought and action.

It is very important that you seize and retain control of your habits and the best way to do this is to start recognizing the influences that you let affect you, the positive ones, shed the negative or destructive ones and regain your own personal power.

You can do this.

Miscommunication

Let's give you an example of language and how miscommunication can happen.

Have you ever tried to communicate with someone who didn't speak your language and they couldn't understand you? A classic example of this is when on holiday when someone goes out to a restaurant in a foreign country and they think they ordered a nice rump steak, but when the food shows up it turns out they actually asked for fish stew.

This is the kind of relationship that most of us have with our own unconscious mind. We might think we are "ordering up" more money, a happy, healthy relationship, peace with our family members, and being able to stick to a healthy diet...but unless this keeps showing up, something is probably getting lost in the language translation.

 NLP we have a saying: the conscious mind is the goal setter and the unconscious mind is the goal getter. Your unconscious mind is not out to get you, rather it's out to get what you want more of in your life.

Try this example right now. If there was one thing you would like to change right now, ust one habit, that you would like to break, what would it be?

- Would you like to remain relaxed during work presentations?
- Stop procrastinating and spending too much time on social media?
- Not eating a whole packet of biscuits once you have opened them?

As we have said before the brain does not understand negative thinking, so you just get more of what you really don't want. However, if you don't know how to communicate what you want properly, it will keep bringing steaming bowls of fish stew out of the kitchen.

In NLP (there is something called the Representational System which examines how you receive and interpret information.

Representational Systems Test – What's your learning style

Good communication depends upon knowing how people's brains are wired. One of the first things that I do when I'm teaching is to identify the way my students take in and process information. I can then build on this to maximise the effectiveness of my work with them. Neuro Linguistic Programming (

There are four representational sensory channels we use to experience and understand our world – visual, auditory (hearing), auditory digital (logical thinking) and kinaesthetic (emotions, touch and bodily sensations). In addition, we make sense of our experiences and understanding in words.

All of our memories, imagination and current experiences are made up of elements of these four "representational systems".

This simple test will allow you to discover your own preferences.

After reading the next few pages, you will:

• Understand about the four different ways people receive and store information.

• Know how you are wired – something that is key for weight loss

• Be able to recognise how other people are wired and understand people more.

• Be able to see, feel, hear or think the best way that you take in information

• Realise how important it is to know how your family and colleagues are wired as well.

Score yourself between 1- 4.

4 points being closest description of you and 1 being the least close description of you.

1. I make important decisions based on:

_____ gut level feelings (K)

_____ which way sounds the best (A)

_____ what looks best to me (V)

_____ precise review and study of the issues (Ad)

2. During an argument I am most likely to be influenced by:

_____ whether or not I am in touch with the other person's point of view (K)

_____ the other person's tone of voice (A)

___whether or not I can see the other person's point of view (V)

_____ the logic of the other person's argument (Ad)

3. I most easily communicate what is going on with me by:

_____ the feelings I share (K)

_____ the tone of my voice (A)

_____ the way I dress and look (V)

_____ the words I choose (Ad)

4. When I am setting up my TV room or living space, it is most important to me to:

_____ select the most comfortable furniture (K)

____ have the sound system set-up so I can play music (A)

_____ have the right colours in the room (V)

_____make sure everything is put in its proper place (Ad)

5. I find that:

_____ I am very sensitive to other people's feelings (K)

_____ I am very aware of the sounds of my surrounding (A)

____ I easily notice changes in the way places or people look (V)

__ I am adept at making sense of new facts and data (Ad)

6. In order to know if someone is doing a good job I need to:

____do the job with them or experience some aspect of their job (K)

____listen to a description of the way they are doing their work (A)

_____see them do the job (V)

____have the facts & figures on the work that has been done (Ad)

7. I find that when I'm at college or a work presentation, I take most notice of information that:

_____ I can learn by doing an activity or exercise (K)

____I can hear, such as what the presenter is saying (A)

___I can see, such as slides, white board or pictures (V)

_____ is presented in terms of facts and figures (Ad)

Add up your total score for each of the letters and add them up below to give you a score which corresponds with your representational system preferences.

The highest score indicates the most significant way with which you deal with, store and take in information and communicate to others.

This is a rough guide to what each representational system means

Visual (V) – Seeing

"Visual" people are most likely to:

- Memorise by seeing pictures
- Have trouble remembering verbal instructions
- Tend to stand up straight, breathe from the top of the chest
- Prefer to stand back so they can see you
- Interested in whether things 'look good'
- Tend to move, think and talk faster

Usually those who have a visual preference will be nicely dressed and well-groomed and their desk will be tidy as they don't like clutter.

Auditory (A) – Hearing

"Auditory" people are most likely to:

- Learn by listening
- Can repeat things back to you easily
- Breathe from middle of chest
- Tone of voice very important
- Interested in whether things 'sound right'
- Like to be close enough to hear you

Easily distracted by noise – I used to work in an office with designers, and we had a constant battle over the radio. They kept turning it up and I kept turning it down because it interfered with the auditory processing I was following in order to get my report to "sound" right.

Kinaesthetic (K) – Feeling

"Kinae" people are most likely to:

- Talk and breathe slowly
- Respond to physical rewards and touch
- Memorise by doing or walking through things
- Breathe from the abdomen
- Interested in whether things 'feel right'
- Like to be close enough to touch you

They will dress for comfort rather than looks. They will probably arrange their office so that everything is in easy reach, even if it looks untidy – they won't even be aware of that unless it's pointed out to them.

Auditory Digital (Ad) - Internal dialogue

"Auditory Digital" people are most likely to:

- A lot of internal dialogue
- Memorise by steps, procedures, sequences
- Interested in whether something 'makes sense'
- Can exhibit characteristics of other systems
- Will often be leaning back (dissociated)

Auditory digital people will likely manifest characteristics of the other 3 representational systems. In addition, they will talk to themselves a lot and like to make sense of things and understand them.

What does understanding representation systems have to do with weight loss ?

For example – if you were to say "I must go running" this does not set up an imaginary picture or an auditory prompt in your brain.

However, if you were to say "I look forward to running in the park, listening to the birds and enjoying the bright sunshine" Now you are building a stronger image in your mind.

The more you build into your representational systems the more you are empowered by the energy you are creating to your weight loss.

When, make your images colourful with nice smells maybe even tastes - and really begin to feel them. This is a very powerful tool you are now learning.

Further NLP information or training can be found on my website. www.garysellors.com

Auto-suggestion Exercise

This lovely exercise will only take a few minutes so you can do this a few times a day, it's best if you close your eyes for a few moments - so please do not do it whilst driving!

"I feel calm. I feel relaxed. I feel in control. As my muscles relax, a beam of sunlight enters through an imaginary opening in the top of my head, like a gentle, warm flow of powerful energy throughout my body.. it removes all my negative thoughts and feelings.. leaving me with only positive thoughts and feelings.. I am calm.... I am relaxed.. I am in control"

"My subconscious mind is now open to receive the helpful and very beneficial suggestions I'm about to give myself."

"I feel really good about my commitment to losing 1 ½ - 2 ½ lbs each week"

"Overeating is like a poison in my body and I don't need that"

"I am in complete control of my eating habits"

"I am now eating more appropriately"

"I love myself and that's a good starting place"

Target shooting

When losing weight certain barriers crop up. n this chapter we will look at how we can remove them one at a time. Look at the list of behavioural changes below and think through how difficult you would find them on a scale of 1 to 10, with the most difficult being 10 and the easy ones being 1. You may find that you are already successfully doing some of these with your new healthy weight loss lifestyle, so if this is the case- WELL DONE and leave them out.

What I would like you to do is to choose one behaviour to which you will commit. You may want to have a go at the toughest ones first; you will then find the others easier - it would be harder the other way round. Once you have completed the first one, start on the next one.

- Eat one more serving of fresh vegetables and fruit a day.
- Replace bad fats (e.g., cheese, biscuits) with good fats (e.g. olive oil).
- Reduce your portion size by a third.
- Stop having second helpings.
- Increase your exercise regimen by an extra a week.
- Eat one less take away per month.
- Replace sugary drinks and other tempting drinks with water.
- Buy a healthy cook book and learn to cook a new dish.
- Remove all unhealthy snacks (e.g. crisps, cakes, sweets) from your cupboards.

- Join a sports centre or gym class.

- For a week really focus on thinking positive and nothing else.

- Set a cut-off time for late night snacks and stick to it.

- Increase the amount of good quality sleep you get.

- Go for a walk at lunch time and or least leave your desk.

- Cook *everything* in olive oil.

- Skip desserts or replace sugary deserts with fruit or healthier options.

Each day make it your mission to change one thing. At the very least, achieve 3 good changes per week let's not forget, YOU ARE IN CONTROL OF YOUR WINNING MIND SET.

You will find once you take that step and start believing that you can make these changes for the better you will begin to feel amazing and just wish you had started earlier.

The voice of negativity

Most of us, if we are honest, have a little bit of weight around our tummies that we could do without. Maybe we have had it since our childhood. Perhaps when we were at school - those good old days - we would "Fatty", "who eats all the pies?" and "Piglet" plus many other names and phrases I'm sure some of you can remember. When I was young I wore glasses and I remember being verbally abused on a daily basis. I would go home and cry, although I would not tell my parents. And then, the next day, I had to go back to school to repeat the process. The joys of school!

Such constant experience of negativity would lead us into low self-esteem, depression and low self-image. Sadly many people remain affected by their childhood experiences. It's amazing how still affect us so much and is much more common than you realize. You are not alone in this thinking.

Let's look at the way we think about exercise and what we think when we miss a session for whatever reason. Listen to what you tell yourself. "I'm useless, I will always be fat", "I will never achieve my weekly planned exercise targets". Think back to what we talked about where your control is and start to be very aware of how you talk to yourself. Most of the talk is going to be negative.

This negative self-talk, is a common area for people reaching for the extra food. Most tummy related problems, in my opinion, have an emotional attachment to them. One way you may look at it is that the extra weight we are carrying becomes something of a protective barrier.

If you think about your personal space and that barrier around you, you start to understand this more plus the more the negative aspects of our self-talk increase, the more you eat and the endless cycle goes on.

The easiest way to deal with and start to change this, is to become aware of what you are saying and when you are saying it. Once you are more aware of your thinking, you can then start challenging it with questions like "What do I gain by thinking this way" or "What is the opposite of my negative thinking". You will be very surprised by the answers you hear. Go with what comes to mind because if you deny it, this won't help you.

Once you have a better understanding of these voices, you can start to replace them with more positive statements and affirmations. Many people who have weight loss issues find that they are linked with low self-esteem, so maybe doing the mirror exercise as discussed in previous chapters is an excellent way of restoring your confidence again.

Here are just a few examples of how you can change your self-talk so that it works for, not against, towards you losing weight.

Negative Self-Talk	Positive Self-Talk
I have no willpower.	To achieve weight loss. I need to act positive not just use willpower. By identifying my habits, planning ahead and thinking positively, I am now achieving my weight loss target.
My mother and father are both overweight. Therefore I will always be fat because it's in my genes.	My genes aren't my destiny. I know I can lose weight with healthier habits.
I'm a hopeless failure. It's been over a week, and I haven't lost a pound.	I may not have lost weight but I did exercise and plan my meals. If I keep making these small changes, I will succeed in my goals.

It's time for my daily punishment for being fat. I have to go to the gym.	Once I finish exercising, I always feel re-energized and in control. love running; it makes me feel wonderful.
It's not fair that I have to eat diet food when everyone else can eat what they want.	Lots of people are watching what they eat. I'm not alone in choosing healthy, nutritious food that my body deserves.
Life is no fun when I'm on a diet.	I make my own fun through friends and activities. Food is only fuel for my body.

I'm a big fan of the phrase *"fake it, till you make it"*. When I suggest the idea that my clients think themselves thin, they look at me after looking at their large tummies and say, *"real world, I'm fat"*. There is much research and science to say that thinking negative thoughts can be a self-filling prophecy and the thinking positively can produce the same results.

The more I learn about neuroscience and understanding the mind I find that when we think of something, it will produce an emotion based on what we are thinking at that moment and this will lead us to react in a certain manner i.e. Thoughts become feelings which then lead to actions.

Most clients laugh when I ask them to imagine themselves as thin. It can take a few goes to starting thinking this way. As I have said before, if you see it in your mind, the brain will believe that it is true, because the brain cannot understand negatives.

From now on always be aware of your positive thinking and the healthy choices that you are making. Remain positive in your thoughts towards your exercises. Keep saying over and over "I love exercising"; "I am losing weight easily and effortlessly"; "I love my body and I love myself all is well". Please go with these; they do work and remember, you have to fake it till you make it. Give it a go - you will love the results.

Just before we finish this chapter, if and when you have a , don't give yourself a hard time. Remember those voices and the control you now have. Please never forget, we are all only human and if you fancy a chocolate or a cake eat it, as you are more likely to keep thinking about it all day if you don't. Just don't eat the whole cake. Tell yourself that you are in control and that you will do it differently next time; perhaps you will not even bring them into the house. Therefore you have adjusted your strategy to helping you lose weight.

The negative self-talk won't be changed over night and it will be hard at first. But as you practice each day, it will get easier and soon you will start to see yourself in a new light with some very positive thinking.

Well done you.

Remember this – You would not talk to your best friend in the way you talk to yourself nor would you give your friend such a hard time. So start to be nicer to yourself.

Apple or pear

Let's look at your waist and the concerns you may need to be aware of. Although you notice that your waist is not changing shape, maybe it's time to have a closer look at what may be going on. It's important to keep an eye on your waist, even if your scales show that you haven't lost any weight.

As we know, in the hot weather our bodies do expand. What people don't realise is that when we are under stress, which affects the stress hormones, the result is that fat accumulates around your midsection. When you feel tension as well, it will have the same effect on your body.

Most people are apple-shaped or pear-shaped. This means that when you put on weight, the fat is either stored around your hips (pear-shaped) or around your middle (apple-shaped).

If you're overweight and apple-shaped, you have a higher risk of health problems than if you're pear-shaped.

An expanding waistline is a warning sign about our overall health. Unlike fat in the thighs or in the hips abdominal fat increases the risk of type 2 diabetes, high blood pressure, high cholesterol and metabolic syndrome - a combination of high levels of cholesterol and blood sugar. This leads to our being overweight and increases our blood pressure.

The best way to measure your waist circumference is to place a tape measure around your bare abdomen. Make sure it is just above your hipbone. Also, make sure the tape measure is tight but does not pinch the skin. Be relaxed and not rushed when measuring and exhale as well.

To measure your waist: (NHS Guidelines)

- find the bottom of your ribs and the top of your hips
- breathe out naturally
- wrap a tape measure around your waist midway between these points to find your measurement

You have a higher risk of health problems if your waist size is:

- more than 94cm (37 inches) if you're a man
- more than 80cm (31.5 inches) if you're a woman

Your risk of health problems is even higher if your waist size is:

- more than 102cm (40 inches) if you're a man
- more than 88cm (34.5 inches) if you're a woman

Most people who are overweight can blame their excess weight on eating more calories than they burn.

Weight gain occurs when we regularly put more calories (energy) into our bodies than we use. Over time, that excess energy is stored by the body as fat. If you're trying to lose weight, it's a good idea to eat less and be more active. If you don't, then you run the serious risk of health consequences such as heart disease.

Why are there separate measurements for Asian men and women?

People of Asian backgrounds tend to have a higher proportion of body fat to muscle than the rest of the UK population. They also tend to carry this fat around the middle. This leads to a greater risk of developing problems such as diabetes and coronary heart disease at a lower waist size than other people in the UK.

- more than 90cm (about 35.5 inches) if you're a man
- more than 80cm (about 31.5 inches) if you're a woman

What is your BMI and how do you change it?

In today's world there is an ever increasing risk of obesity. Some figures point to the fact that 30% of the population in the UK are . This in itself is putting a massive strain on the body and the UK health service as they try and tackle the issues. Understanding what a healthy body should be has never been more important.

Conditions that can be related to obesity can affect your Body Mass Index (BMI). In western countries it is considered that 90% of type 2 diabetes cases are caused by being very overweight. Being overweight has always been linked with increases in heart disease and strokes.

The World Cancer Research Fund (WCRF) wrote a report which reflected that having a healthy body weight of (BMI of 20-25) was one of the main key issues in the prevention of cancer (October 2007).

Let's look at BMI in more detail and from a practical point of view so that you will be able to understand what it is and how you can work out your own BMI. Knowing your BMI puts you in a stronger position to be in control of your body and make changes if and when needed. To begin with you need to know your weight in kilograms and height in metres. Most modern scales that we can buy now show weight in kilograms. The use of a calculator or various websites or even apps makes it easy for you to work out your BMI.

The Body Mass Index was developed by the World Health Organisation. This is a simple height/weight ratio which enables people to quickly and easily work out if they are over or under weight or even obese.

Follow this example for working out your BMI. Take your weight in kilograms divided by the square of your height in meters (kg/m²). For example, an adult who weighs 70kg who is 1.75m tall will have a BMI of 22.9.

$$BMI = \frac{70 \ (kg)}{1.75^2 \ (m^2)} = 22.9 \ (kg/m^2)$$

The BMI scores show that where you are:

- Under 20 you are considered to be underweight
- Between 20 and 25 you are a normal weight
- Between 25 and 30 you are overweight
- Between 30 and 35 you are obese
- Above 35 you are clinically obese.

There will always be the . That some people have larger muscle .Therefore affect their BMI; sports players would be an example of this where the weight gain is due to muscle enhancement. I always say to my clients, if you *FEEL* overweight then you are. It's about time you did something about it. You don't really need BMI and other measurements. These are just healthy guidelines that shouldn't be ignored.

How much weight should come off?

Let's look at what you can now do to reduce your size and empower you to lower your BMI. Let's say your height is 1.8 m and you weigh 90 kg; your BMI is 27.7 which is overweight. To bring this down to a healthier weight you would probably choose to increase your exercise and improve what you eat. So that brings the question, what weight should you aim for?

Really feeling very inspired having read this far into the book and being able to take control, you might decide that you want to get to a healthy BMI of 22. Using this information, you can calculate that to achieve a BMI of 22 you need to get your weight down to 71.5kg (22/27.7) x 90 kg = 71.5 kg.

Use this very useful tool from the NHS.uk website

www.nhs.uk/Tools/Pages/Healthyweightcalculator

A little reminder, to show your understanding so far.

Let's look at how well you are doing with what you have read so far, in this book. The more you understand weight loss now, the more successful you will be in achieving you goal. Here is a little test for you. It is only a guideline to show you the weight loss journey you are on. There is no right and wrong – this is just an indication of what you have achieved so far.

1. I don't sit down for more than an hour as I now get up and move about. I do this whether I'm at work or on my day off. Any movement is good for me.

2. I now use more positive affirmation techniques as discussed in this book Which keeps me positive Therefore I remain in control for my eating habits.

3. I am much more conscious of what I am putting in my mouth when I eat my food.

4. I have reduced my takeaways; no more than one a week.

5. I am more aware of my comfort foods now and I know that after 20 minutes the feeling will pass and I can be proud that I just didn't grab some food.

6. I plan my morning for getting up and exercising with by setting my alarm the night before.

7. If I weigh myself each week I find that my weight has increased, I set out to do more exercise.

8. I now take responsibility for myself and don't blame my genes, family or any other excuse for my weight gain as I used to do in the past.

9. I now enjoy checking out the labels and calorie content of the food I buy on my shopping trips.

10. I am now so much more in control of my thoughts, feelings and actions.

11. I now choose to eat fresh fruit and fresh seasonal vegetables, rather than the crisps, snacks and cakes that I used to eat.

12. I now choose to take control of my voices in my head and I choose which thoughts that I will listen to.

13. I am more aware of portion sizes and aim to drink at least 2 litres of water each day.

14. I am learning more and enjoying this book as I go on my weight loss journey.

How did you get on with the little reminder? If you can only agree with a few comments so far no worries. This highlights the work that needs to be done. Most clients I work with find that the reminder is a refresh of the book so far and some often say that they didn't realise how much they had now learned.

Review this reminder about once a month; put a mark in your diary and monitor your successful progress. Keep up the great work.

Writing your thoughts down

Let's look at the emotional eating side of weight loss. This is linked with consuming large amounts of food because we have an emotional attachment more than we realise sometimes. At times we just respond to food as a way of helping us through emotional upsets.

Sometimes we make excuses to reach for foods that make us happy - and then later we regret having eaten it.. There is much research to say that our emotions are linked with over eating. Therefore weneed to learn new strategies and other ways of coping.

A good idea is to make a note and keep a record of thoughts, feelings and actions over a time period. Clients often find that writing about these areas can have a positive effect on mental and physical health.

Keeping a diary of your thoughts, feelings and actions are proven way to successful weight loss. As previously noted this creates a good manual of your life and enables you to review what works and what doesn't and highlights the many successes you have had.

It is important to remember that this is not a food diary but about the thoughts and feelings which create the emotional imbalance. This psychological assessment affects your underlying emotions which will, once on paper in front of you, empower you to dealing with each emotion as the need arises.

When you start this recording of your thoughts and feelings it's important to set aside time to do this correctly. Remember that this in itself is another example of how you are now more in control of your life, thanks to all the work you have done so far in the book. Decide what time would be best for you.

Some clients like to do this at the end of the day, some at lunchtime and others at a coffee break; it works better if you put a time scale to it as well, maybe 20 minutes.

The key to maximising the effectiveness of this exercise is doing the work in a calm and relaxed manner and not finding excuses. Remember, you don't have to write something every day though I would recommend that you do at least 3 days a week.

An example of your journal could look like this

My Journal	Thoughts	Feelings	Emotions
Emotional outbursts			
Social			
Situation			

Some areas of concern for your eating triggers could be in these areas.

Thoughts. This could show that you turn to food as a result of negative thinking, maybe linked with your low self-worth, guilt and triggers from the past.

Emotional outbursts. These outbursts could be related to stress, tension at work or family life, depression, anger, anxiety or loneliness that you are currently experiencing or even boredom.

Social. When you are around people, you are encouraged to eat for the sake of eating. This could be because you want to fit in with the crowd, want to impress new friends or maybe you have had an argument or just feeling inadequate.

Situation. This is when you go on holiday and are offered an all you can eat buffet - the food is just there. More and more places are offering food nowadays. Clients who go to the cinema have to buy a bucket of popcorn or those tempting sweets. Sitting in front of the TV is another popular place of temptation for eating snacks for many clients.

Or perhaps you eat to console yourself; you tell yourself that its your only pleasure whereas the really constructive action would be to tackle the problem that drives you to seek consolation.

Maybe other situations are triggers for you. When you start keeping this record of your thoughts and emotions as you eat you will be surprised by some of the things that come up.

Another way of recording your thoughts and feelings is a technique called *reflection*. Reflection requires us to think through what has happened and think why or how something took place/was said etc. We can add in what alternatives we might have tried/said etc. This is most effective when you write it as a form of journal or blog; some people find it easier to written the third person.

An example of this would be:

"As she walked to work, looking down on the ground, saying to herself that she will just eat the snacks in her office drawer when she gets to work and this has really got to stop".

This time she will talk to her office colleagues about other ways of losing weight for encouragement."

Another good suggestion is to have a dialogue between 2 people where you are both people. Some people like to see this as the good and the bad person in you; this can be really fun, very honest and always interesting. An idea is to have 2 bits of paper, headed up good and other bad list the benefits of both and then discuss what you have written with yourself. What you may find is that at some point in this exercise there will be an understanding that a middle ground can be reached.

This in itself can be very powerful. If you become stuck repeat what you have just written and add the word… Because…….

This will open up your thinking.

Then work with what comes up. This is a very powerful chapter, it may bring up some emotions which may surprise you and at times might upset you and cause you to shed a tear. If it gets too heavy, work with a friend. Or another great tip that works well for my clients is to write what has come up on paper as quickly as you can. DO NOT READ IT. Just write.

Then hrow the piece of paper away; burn it or just rip it up. This is a very empowering exercise.

By doing this, those thoughts and feelings that surfaced are gone and very much in the past. Well done you; you have worked hard today.

Having a supportive network

When losing weight, it is an extra benefit if you have a supportive structure around you. This could be in the form of a friend, partner, husband, wife, coffee group, social network or friends. There is much research to say that when the support you receive is positive then your journey of weight loss is fun.

There can be people, who once you start losing weight get . You may find that friends change and don't like the success you are having. You will be surprised how some can become quite jealous. This will be because, although they appeared in the beginning to support you, really they were thinking "it won't last"; "it's only a ". However, you have shown that your life is changing for the better.

Friends may start to think that because you are changing and losing weight successfully that you will not like them anymore and that you will seek or more like minded people. Don't be surprised when you hear comments, like "you're doing so well let's celebrate and have a cake as a reward" or "you look fine as you are: don't lose any more weight".

The good thing about this when it happens, which it will do, is that you will have become much more in control of the choices and will be more prepared when these comments and green eyed monsters come your way. You will be ready to deal with them in a calm manner with a massive smile on your face.

Let's look at the positive side of having good support. It involves people that you can trust and who can help you on your journey. The help you get can vary in so many different ways. It could be a simple preparing healthy food for you when you are going to work or running late. This gives you love and support and indicates an understanding of what you are now aiming for.

Maybe it comes in the form of having someone look after the children while you attend your gym class or weight loss session group or someone who teaches the children to wash up after dinner /lunchtime so that you don't hang around the kitchen eating scraps. This way you avoid the kitchen and temptation.

It's nice when you discuss losing weight at work and you find that some other people want also to lose weight and don't have the confidence that you now have. Then work colleagues might suggest going for a lunchtime walk, which over time increases in distance. You may be surprised to that other people want to join this positive group. Positivity always attracts Positivity.

Stages of change for exercise

As discussed in early chapters about changing behaviours. We adapt this exercise to know and learn more about exercising for a healthier lifestyle, by changing our behaviour.

It states that at any time, for any behaviour, individuals are at one of the following six stages of behaviour change:

Pre-contemplation (not active and not thinking about becoming active)

The person is unlikely to be aware that they have a problem to address. At this stage to have no desire to make any changes and is not the least bit interested in being different. Their time scale is. Nothing is wrong or everything is just fine and in a year's time everything will still be just fine. some people around us may think we have a problem or are showing concern for us but we don't agree with their concern and say things like "there is nothing wrong with me". From a weight loss journey that you own, this would mean that you are comfortable with your weight, exercise levels and health. This can be classed as being in denial.

Contemplation (not active but thinking about becoming active)

The important part about this stage is the thinking about it although sadly thinking doesn't use any calories. Some clients like to think back to what sports they use to enjoy - riding a bike, ice skating, playing football or netball. Look at the pros and cons about starting up new sports again they will not seem as bad as you make out.

At this contemplation stage we tend to start to think that there may be a problem and that we should start to maybe do something about it. It can sometimes be the little things like a shortage of breath when you walk or those clothes that you haven't worn for while seem a little tighter.

These are very much tell-tale signs. Once they recognize that something was not what it was like before clients then start in this "wishing things were different stage" "*I wish I was thin*". "*I wish I could be fitter*". From this thinking, clients fall into the SHOULD DO category. "I should lose weight", "I should go to the gym". "*I should do a lot of things*"

Commitment (decide that you have to become active)

At this stage it's all about clients making a decision because they now admit that they have a problem and the good thing is that they are now motivated to make a difference to their bodies and their unhealthy lifestyles. Their health may be at risk and they start saying things that are very negative. "We don't like ourselves" and "we have had enough" and "things have got worse and need to change". What happens now is that we go from "*I* " to saying things like "I will change". This is not an easy stage to get to; sometimes the pain or unhappiness is still not enough just yet. It always amazes me how low people will go before they get to this commitment stage. Rest assured you will reach this stage sooner or later.

Preparation (active but not at recommended levels)

The key is to identify specific barriers that you think limit your ability to losing weight and exercising more. An example would be that you like to run in the summer but in the winter it's wet and cold. So what other choices have you in place such that you can run all year round? Preparation is the key to this stage.

It's often recommended that you keep a record of what is going on, the type of workout you do, the length of your exercise time etc. Just as with your eating, note the exercise you take and the time of day (morning etc) and how you felt during and after the session. You will be able to analyse the most productive exercise schedule for you. Also, as you look back you will see how far you have come and, being aware of how much fitter you are now, your motivation to continue will be maintained – and probably increase.

The good thing here is that you have decided to change. The mind set in your head is so much more positive now. You are so much more in control now. Because you are now recording what you are doing with your exercise routine, you can begin to see what works and what doesn't, and you are better informed to identify and implement the changes that need to be made.

When you are stuck on certain changes do some brain storming. Get out some paper and a pen and just write down all the mad, crazy things that come into your mind about the changes that you could make.

Once you have a train of thought you mind starts rolling and you will be surprised by what great ideas can come up. You will start moving things that could lead us backwards; cupboards full of snacks, old trainers, anything that could stop us now in our preparation tracks for the positive future of change.

Action (active at recommended levels for less than six months)

Now you are changing your routines because you are really enjoying this stage. For many clients it can be a light bulb moment. You are now in great place, physically and emotionally. This stage can be a spiritual awakening that leads to a better life.

This stage is so much about you and about you being in control and if and when things need to be changed you now make the right decisions, the right positive choices. You will see the clear path ahead which is the spiritual path. You now enjoy being in control and the secret is to keep this up, as most people know if you do something for more than 21days, it then becomes a habit. That's all it takes to trigger a better life.

Maintenance (just doing what you do best) Lose weight

You are now at the final stage of just maintaining and very much aware of the plateau after 6-8 weeks. S prepared for this, because you know it i was going to happen. .The body adapts and normalises it . So maintaining change is excellent for you and your weight loss plan.

It's proven that to get the best results keep the brain guessing what you are going to do next. It's a known fact in neuroscience that if you don't give the brain something to do it starts going backwards and using old thinking. It has been shown that people who are in a position to maintain healthy changes for a minimum of six months have shown to be more successfully in reaching their goals.

"An average person with average talent, ambition and education, can outstrip the most brilliant genius in our society, if that person has clear, focused goals".

Brian Tracy

What do the scales say to you? - Who is in control

We all know that you carefully stand on and talk to?, or sneak up them?, lean to one side of them to keep your weight . But the scales know what you're up to.

Let's look at different ways you could approach your scales and make them friendlier. It all comes to the way you see the result. It is always best to be real about what you see on the scales; then you can address the issues.

That's it weight - Meaning you have had enough and are never going back to that weight. It's the weight argument you make with yourself that you are are not prepared to accept this anymore. Enough is enough!

Fed up weight - Just looking at the weight figure makes you feel fed up and that has a knock-on effect with your state of mind.

That's acceptable weight – It's not good or bad, just that you accept it as the way it is. It's good to note that can work for and against you as some clients get too comfortable and don't realise that the weight creeps up into fed up weight. *Just be careful.*

That's good news weight – You are heading in the right direction and that's good news. It is still not the final result but you are now very much on course with what you're working towards. Keep it up.

Target weight – This is what you have always wanted and worked so hard to achieve, some see it as a dream weight.

As discussed in previous chapters, let's look again at writing down what you think about the different weight categories and look at addressing the difference between your real weight and your fed up weight.

How do you feel about it? What are you going to do next? What changes in your exercise routine are you going to make? Discuss with trusted friends and make notes. This session is always good for a bit of brain storming and can be fun while you do it.

When you reach your target weight make sure you have strategies in place to maintain the new healthy future and confident you in place.

Another point to remember is whatever the number is, it is really important about what you think about your size because you are not just a number. You are a loving person who is now in control of your own thoughts and feelings.

Keep up the good work – You can succeed.

Lose the cravings with EFT (That tapping thing)

EFT is very easy to learn, and will help you:

- Remove Negative Emotions
- Reduce Food Cravings
- Reduce or Eliminate Pain
- Set Positive Goals

EFT (Emotional Freedom Technique) is a form of psychological based on the same energy meridians used in traditional acupuncture to treat physical and emotional ailments for over five thousand years but without the invasiveness of needles. Instead, simple tapping with the fingertips is used to input kinetic energy onto specific meridians on the head and chest while you think about your specific problem. It works very well with traumatic events, addictions, pain, etc.

This combination of tapping the energy meridians and voicing positive affirmation works to clear the emotional blocks around you achieving your weight loss and thus restoring your mind and body's balance.

Some people are initially wary of the principles underlying EFT: The electromagnetic energy that flows through the body and regulates our health has only recently started to become recognized. Others are initially taken aback (and sometimes amused) by the EFT tapping and affirmation methodology.

This EFT script will help you with your cravings for food, sweets and other cravings that stop you losing weight. I use for helping people to stop smoking.

All you have to do to adapt this script is to replace the word craving with what your addiction is.

- It is very important that you have a level of intensity towards the craving to start with. 0 = no craving, 10 = you must have it

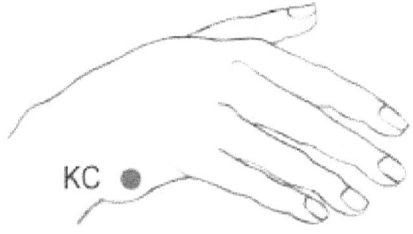

KC

- Repeat this affirmation 3 times, while tapping on the Karate chop (KC) point

"Even though I have this craving, I deeply and profoundly love and accept myself"

"Even though I have this craving, I deeply and profoundly love and accept myself"

"Even though I have this craving, I deeply and profoundly love and accept myself"

- Now begin tapping with your fingertips, 10 times on each point. Focus on your craving and keep repeating the reminder phrase at each tapping point.

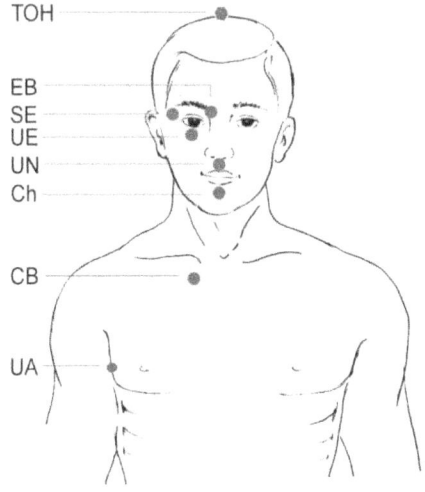

The Tapping points:-

1. Top of the Head: "This craving, I must have it now"

2. Eyebrow: "This craving is all I can think about   at present"

3. Outside of Eye: "This craving is starting to drive me mad"

4. Under your Eye: "This craving, I need it now"

5. Under your Nose: "This craving, I feel useless"

6. Chin: "This craving, I can feel the emotions"

7. Collar Bone: "This craving, Isn't who I am"

8. Under Arm: "This craving, I am now letting go"

Now, Take a deep breath and exhale slowly

Now review your original starting number of the craving. Has it gone down now or has it disappeared?

At this point, you will find that things are starting to change and the intensity of your craving is now starting to reduce in numbers. If you still feel the craving is the exactly the same, no worries. This does happen now and then. Just start again with the tapping points above. Just before you start again. Tap on the Karate Chop (KC) 50 times it doesn't matter which hand you use.

If the craving intensity has gone down from your last number, just repeat the process and focus on the lower number and craving. Keep repeating this until the cravings and number have got down to 1 or zero.

Medical Professionals comments:

Bruce Lipton, PhD
"EFT is a simple, powerful process that can profoundly influence gene activity, health and behavior."

Deepak Chopra, MD
"EFT offers great healing benefits."

Dr Mercola, MD (bestselling author and health commentator in US)
"The Emotional Freedom Technique, or EFT, is the psychological acupressure technique I routinely use in my practice and most highly recommend to optimize your emotional health. Although it is still often overlooked, emotional health is absolutely essential to your physical health and healing - no matter how devoted you are to the proper diet and lifestyle, you will not achieve your body's ideal healing and preventative powers if emotional barriers stand in your way."

Note: Once you have got comfortable with the EFT process and tapping on yourself you can use it to tap on other people, which can be fun. Also, if you just think about the tapping points and where you tap, it will work just the same. So you can be standing at a bus stop, in a meeting or sitting on the toilet. It all works. I have worked with children and EFT and I have them bring a comfort toy and I teach them to tap on teddy. This proves that it all comes from the intention you put into this exercise.

For more information about EFT and its many uses I would recommend Gary Craig's original site www.emofree.com I have spent many years learning, training and watching all the available DVDs.

Negative thinking – Stop it

In this chapter I would like to look more closely at our thoughts and how they affect you, which then has a knock-on effect on your success in relation to your weight loss journey. The more we understand neuroscience, the more people are now realising that what you think does affect your body.

A lot of clients tend to think that the success of weight loss is one thing or the other, often complete opposites (e.g. all or nothing), almost like your being two different people. In this mode of thinking there is never any middle ground; it's as clear as black and white in their thinking process. An example of this would be that if you have gained 2 lbs and with negative thinking this means that you will never achieve your weight loss; the reverse would be that if you lost 3lbs you feel you could conquer the world.

What's important to remember is that the weighing scales don't tell the full story as extra weight gain could be linked with water retention or illness; for example, when we are ill we tend not to eat so therefore lose weight. With this thinking process we can forget these things and how it impacts on the body.

Emotional thought processes are where you are guided by your feelings rather than your thoughts. But remember - thoughts affect feelings first. So when you say you "don't feel like exercising" or "I'm not in the mood for a salad", Go back to your brain and in charge of your thinking your thinking and notice how you start to feel.

The intuitive side of me is used to a bit of fortune telling. When I hear clients saying things like "I don't think I will ever lose weight" or "I predict that I will always be fat" the best way I find to advise them in how to deal with this type of thinking is by asking them to clarify their goals, often best expressed in picture form.

Have them look at some old photos of themselves being happy and smiling and place these pictures on your vision board, or on the fridge or kitchen door. Place a photo somewhere you will see it every day in your psyche and let it feed into your subconscious mind. This works very well and yet you don't notice it.

Have you ever notice that when you just focus on one thing, you seem to see it everywhere; an example, you notice a purple car pass you and from then . You start to see them everywhere, or if you see a pregnant , then everyone seems to be pregnant and yet before you never noticed these things.
Another way of thinking is blaming everything and making it personal. An example of this would be *"Its raining; I can't go running"* . Sounds like an excuse to me. *"When I used to come home from school, if I did my homework, my Mum would give me a large cake ... and that's why I'm fat"* .

Let us face the real facts here in the very practical world of advising about weight loss. GET OVER IT........ and go running in the rain. OK you will get wet: So what? It can be fun and as a good friend used to say to me "we are not made of sugar".

The lesson to learn here is that the quicker you take responsibility for your life and your weight loss the quicker you will succeed.

A little phrase I often say to people. We have two choices if you don't like something: either **change it** or **accept it but don't** sit on the fence and keep moaning about it.

Lastly, Let us look at what happens when you have eaten a lovely large chocolate cake. Now you feel you have blown your whole diet plans. When you step back and just listen to yourself, is it really the end of the world? Is one large chocolate cake going to end it all? Remember you are now in control so remain in control of your thinking.

This week listen carefully to how you think and what you are saying to yourself with your internal voices. When you hear yourself giving yourself a hard time, or catch yourself being self-defeating. Stop the voices; change . Take your mind off automatic pilot and when this happens challenge yourself to think more logically.

A Little Fun Exercise

Try this – Fold your arms across your chest as you would normally. Notice how comfortable you feel and happy. Now release them and fold your arms the other way, the way that you never do as it doesn't feel right. Notice how uncomfortable and very different this feels. It is so much easier to do it the normal way the way you have always done.

Now release and fold them the uncomfortable way again. This time, as you hold them across your chest. Take three deep breaths.

Now release and let go.

Now for a third time, refold your arms in the old uncomfortable way and notice how different and not so uncomfortable this way now feels. This works very well and is all about the breathing that you did and how your body is now getting used to a new you and a new way of folding your arms. You can adapt this exercise in so many ways.

Past YOU Present YOU

This simple little exercise; you will be surprised by the results.

While thinking about why you are overweight list 10 problems/ difficulties you experience by being overweight. may be related to painful memories, particularly as you delve into the reasons behind your list. Be honest with yourself as that is the only way to true progress. e your time

An example would be –

1.   Struggling to get in my clothes

2.   Get stuck in ticket barriers

3.   Walking fast wears you out

4.   Family photos of me are an embarrassment

5.   I don't love myself

6.   I feel rejected

7.   Airplane seats are getting smaller

8.   Chips are my favourite meal

9.   I have no friends

10. I notice people laughing at me as I pass by

List your 10 reasons below:-

1.

2.

3.

4.

5.

6.

7.

8.

9.

10.

Thinking about your life now you have lost the weight, what is good in your life – what do you enjoy?
The examples are of what is great not "how"!

An example would be –

1. Wearing a sexy black number

2. Love running around the park

3. Enjoy the attention I now get from new friends

4. Beach trips are fun and enjoy wearing a bikini

5. I feel sad for other people now, who can't move quickly

6. Having sex is fun again

7. I enjoy feeling amazing and very confident

8. I now notice how much smaller my shopping basket is

9. I love buying new smaller clothes

10. I am so in control now - an amazing feeling

List your 10 reasons below:-

1.

2.

3.

4.

5.

6.

7.

8.

9.

10.

Take a copy of these lists and place them on your food cupboards, secret draws, under the bed boxes, so each time you reach for those comfort foods that make you overweight they are in front of you, challenging your need to eat. You can look at the overweight list then review the success list and then make a choice. As discussed before **You are now in control and have choices.**

Self-hypnosis brings success for weight loss

People are surprised that you can use self-hypnosis for helping you lose weight. This is a little secret gem for you and one that should not be ignored. I have used hypnotherapy for many things over the years and have brought great success to a lot of people

Hypnosis has been around for many years and was known well before people started calorie counting and obsessing about what they were eating. is easy to do and helps you lose weight and - more importantly - keep it off.

Hypnotherapy in 2015 is still not seen by the government as a very successful tool for changing thought patterns and achieving goals, although it is being used more and more by the NHS and other medical centres. It is a shame that the government still does not it. The reason for this seems to be if you cannot see it you cannot show how it is done and hence no evidence (as defined by government). in the future hypnotherapy will get the full credit for the many successes it has achieved.

And of course stage hypnotists have not helped the public perception of hypnotherapy as a serious and beneficial tool.

Due to the lack of research into hypnotherapy. Self-hypnosis has remained a secret for most people. People still struggle to understand how a little mind/body approach can help them with weight loss and build their confidence. Seeing the new you in your mind will, as discussed in previous chapters, have you believing and, more importantly, bring great success into your life.

I have laid out a step by step guide with the weight loss suggestions that I give to my therapy clients using self-hypnosis.

1. You already have the answer within.

Hypnotherapy allows you to go within yourself and succeed and by doing this you then won't need to do crash diets or the latest media hype diet craze. Losing weight is about is about you believing in your own abilities, and then through the power of your mind success will be achieved. Remember when you learned to drive? You thought that you would be able to drive on your own then one day you did. This was because you kept practising and believing that one day you would be able to. Now it's automatic. Losing weight will be the same.

2. See it in your mind will achieve.

You see this so much nowadays in sports athletes. We saw it at the 2012 Olympics and in Formula One. You notice with these examples that when people see something in their mind, they tend to achieve it. This is what using self- hypnosis is about, helping you weight loss.

3. State it in the very positive.

The brain does not understand negatives. Saying things like. "I don't think about cakes any more" just reminds you to focus on cakes. "My body is now healthy and strong in every way". This highlights what you want and in the positive. Avoid negative suggestions. There are many versions of mantras "Unwanted food in my body is not now needed. I'm allowing myself to shed the weight I don't need".

4.   Build it in your mind; see it in your reality.
When you visualise it in your mind, in full colour, with feelings and emotions, (because this makes the image more powerful) it will bring great success. Make your visualization big and colourful, as a child would. You are only limited by your thoughts so dream amazingly. See yourself as a healthy eater Notice what you are wearing, how you are looking. See the healthy foods you now eat. Another way to do this is see a wise old man in a forest / hill top setting who has great advice for you.

5.   A white cloud to take away your cravings.
imagine a large empty cloud floating above your head . You notice a magical cord coming from it and attaching itself to your brain. Now see in your mind all those cravings and wanting food thoughts going up the cord into the large cloud. Feel yourself getting lighter.

Spend a few minutes, releasing all your food thoughts up into the cloud. Notice the cloud getting darker with all that negativity. When you feel that you have let go of all the cravings that are holding you back on your weight loss journey, ut the cord and see the cloud floating away. As this happens you notice in the middle of the cloud is a bright light starting to burn brightly and growing bigger and bigger. All of a sudden the dark cloud explodes into brightness and then it's gone. You are now free.

6.   Be flexible and change it often.

Once you get idea of self- hypnosis the more you will be able to keep changing it and allowing it more flexibility. Let us look at changing the size of what you eat, a notion that works well with people wanting to give up chocolate. See yourself in a closed room all on your own. The walls are made of chocolate; the table and chair also of chocolate.

On the table is a massive pile of chocolate for you to enjoy. You must eat it all. As you eat each piece, it magically reappears so never ending supply of chocolate which you must eat. As you can imagine you start to fill unwell with the amount of chocolate you have eaten, but you must eat it all as you love chocolate. As you can imagine at some point you will say *I DON'T WANT ANYMORE. I HATE CHOCOLATE.* Very few people go back to chocolate after this .. the work is done. Just be flexible with this tool and you will find you can use it in many different.

7.   Practice.

Running around the park once, won't lose all your weight. It is very important that you set time aside to self-hypnosis. This is an amazing tool for you to use to achieve your success. Everyone has heard of the 21 day cycle. Repeat something for 21 days in succession and this will lead you to change your behaviours. Remember also that if you try in one session of self-hypnosis to reduce your weight, stop craving, be confident and increase your exercise it will not work. You would well to focus on just one thing. Keep taking small steps moving forward.

Keep repeating positive affirmations whenever you get a moment.

A great one, Emile Coue, the master of autosuggestion, said "Every day, in every way I am getting better and better" . For weight loss we could change it to

"Every day in every way, I am becoming healthier and loving my new slim body".

"Beautiful, beautiful, beautiful, beautiful boy,
"Before you go to sleep,
"Say a little prayer,
"Every day in every way,
"It's getting better and better."

– John Lennon, *Beautiful Boy (Darling Boy)*, 1980

"Goals that are not written down are just wishes."

Anonymous

Burn calories while you do everyday things

This chapter is about burning calories without knowing that you are already doing it. people think about dieting and losing weight they start to think that they must go the gym and work out as the only way to lose calories. You will be pleasantly surprised how simple housework and gardening also burn calories.

Work done outside in the garden

When in the garden simple tasks like digging, planting and cutting grass burns calories without your noticing this can help tone up muscles in your legs and arms.

Here are some interesting figures:

- Washing the car - good for arms and abdominals and burn 140 calories for every 30 minutes washing.

- When you are digging in the garden for 30 minutes using calves, thighs and shoulders you will burn about 315 calories.

- Going for a nice 45 minute cycle ride with the family uses up 320 calories.

- Doing 30 minutes worth of good old fashion weeding will burn 115 calories; this type of work uses the thighs and buttocks.

- Raking leaves and grass for 30 minutes will use 225 calories.

Indoors work

- Cleaning the bathroom, scrubbing the tiles and cleaning the bath - great arms and shoulders workout, uses 200 calories over 30 minutes.

- Making the beds for 30 burns 130 calories; this can be the equivalent of using the treadmill for 15 minutes on the flat setting.

- Carrying those heavy shopping bags from the supermarket, making sure you use both arms to keep you balanced, not just your strongest arm burns 190 calories if you do it for 30 minutes.

- Time for a spot of window cleaning. Do it for 30 minutes and burn 125 calories.

- Washing dishes for 30 minutes burns will burn 160 calories whereas loading the dishwasher for the same time burns 105.

- When vacuuming the house for 30 minutes you burn 90 calories, the same as boxing for 15 minutes.

- Dusting the house for 30 minutes burns 50 calories.

- Sunday afternoon ironing do it for 30 minutes each week, to burn 70 calories.

- Climbing the stairs for 30 minutes uses 285 calories.

- Painting and decorating your home, will burn 160 calories an hour.

What's eating you?

Emotional eating is about what's eating you. Understand this and the cravings will stop and you will be in a stronger position. We turn to food for comfort, relief and even sometimes as a reward. The reward side can be linked with past events when you have done well and then you have had a reward. Emotional eating doesn't fix emotional problems. It can easily have a negative side and therefore the issue of why we had food remains and you feel guilty for overeating.

The first step is to recognize the triggers of over-eating and what makes you unhappy. Once you start understanding this you will begin to break free from the cravings and this will lead you to changing habits that have sabotaged you in the past.

An example of eating for emotional reasons would be that you have gone out for a nice meal and are already full. Then the dessert menu is brought and you want one! Even though you know you are already full. You tell yourself you have had a bad/busy day/week and deserve a treat.

You give away your control and eat the lot! Did you think about having a low calorie drink instead e.g. a plain coffee or sharing?

People tend to use food as a reward or a pick me up. Now this is all right if you are in control. It only becomes a problem when you have set it as the first port of call - it's a problem if your first impulse when angry, lonely, stressed or bored is too reach for unhealthy foods and this then gets you stuck in a cycle.

Experience will show that filling yourself with foods is not the answer, although it will feel good at that precise moment. Then suddenly after you have eaten you then get the downside and most people will feel worse than they did in the first place. This then leads to beating yourself up for not having enough self-control, so you continue to beat yourself up and the cycle repeats itself. From this you start to feel powerless in respect of what you are eating.

If you are not sure you are an emotional eater or not ask yourself these questions.

- Do you eat more when you're feeling fed up?

- Do you eat when you're not hungry?

- Do you eat when you're not hungry or when you're full?

- Do you eat to feel better (to calm and soothe yourself when you're sad, stressed, anxious, etc.)?

- Do you reward yourself with food at every opportunity?

- Do you regularly eat until you've stuffed yourself?

- Does food make you feel loved?

- Do you feel powerless or out of control around food?

If **"YES"** is the most common response to the above questions, then this highlights that you are eating because of how you **feel** and not what you **need.** Diets may work for you in the short term; however, unless you confront your emotional eating and the hidden motives for over eating they will fail in the longer term.

The danger is that you will revert to your original eating patterns once you have achieved your current weight goal. Since neither emotions nor food ever really go away you have to learn how to deal with both for as long as you live.

We have discussed many ways to regain control within this book. So is nice to have a choice of what you decide will work for you.

Let's look at some of the causes of emotional eating

• **The stuffing down of emotions.** A good practice of dealing with emotions that keep coming up to the surface is have a look at what the body is trying to show you. You will know what it is trying to say. The emotions that may come up could be stress, sadness, anxiety, feeling unloved, fear. When dealing with them don't be surprised if you start crying but once you have let it out you will always feel a lot better.

• **A feeling of loneliness and just being bored.** This is a common one for most people. With the available information technology nowadays people seem even less likely to go out and their social confidence gets knocked. So people find themselves at home on their own and boredom and loneliness start to creep in. People reach for food to fill that emptiness, because it distracts them from the underlying feelings and other distractions.

• **Social influences.** When you get together with family and friends everyone relaxes and enjoys a good time. There is usually plenty of drink and food and before you notice it, all the food is gone. Whilst getting together can be a good way of reducing stress it can sometimes get out of control. When working with weight loss clients I have noticed that clients from certain cultures and backgrounds are expected to attend large family gatherings where they are expected to eat a lot of food. This can be difficult socially especially if people think there is something wrong if you don't eat up – or even take offence. Learn tricks to control yourself; make the best food choices, conceal amounts, not go along with the group and, above all, don't eat too much.

- **The effects of stress.** You will find the more uncontrolled stress you have in your life the more likely you are to turn to emotional eating. There is much research that shows when we are stressed we release Cortisol. which is caused by high levels of the stress hormone. This in turn creates a craving for salty, sweet, high fat foods. What people get from these foods is a burst of energy and pleasure. Once again highlighting that having more control in your life is the key.

*Cortisol is made by the adrenal glands. Cortisol levels go up when the pituitary gland releases another hormone called adrenocorticotropic hormone (ACTH). Cortisol has many functions. It helps the body use sugar (glucose) and fat for energy (metabolism) and it helps the body manage stress.

Once you have identified your true feelings from the triggers you have noticed, look further inside yourself to find the underlying reason. Do you remember the writing exercise that we have discussed before? Do it again now; this will help you a lot and will bring to your conscious mind so you will have a much clearer understanding.

Put your body not your emotions in charge of what you eat. In order to keep your mind and body balanced avoid letting yourself get really hungry and don't starve yourself; this will only lead to you feeling low and trigger a need for extra food.

Some people like to have a treat at the end of the week and as its planned and you're looking forward to it you find that you won't cheat and a have a quick snack, which you know in the longer term won't be rewarding. Also remember the 20 minute exercise; when you're craving for something keep yourself busy for just 20 minutes and the craving will pass.

Let your body feel how you're feeling without eating. A good exercise is when you get a feeling in your body ask yourself what your body is trying to tell you. Once you get your answer, the feeling will go. You will be surprised when you do this, both at how effective it is and by what comes up as the answer.

It's like the saying "we know what is wrong with us, we just need someone to tell us what we already know"

Become Mindful

Mindfulness is very much a topical subject and more people are just beginning to understand how it can help them. Mindfulness is an ancient Asian exercise that involves maintaining awareness in the present moment. Mindfulness keeps us in the here and now state, thinking about what *is* rather than *what if* or *if only.*

The way to start mindfulness is to tune in to each part of your body and begin scanning your body from head to toe. As you do this, notice the difference in the various sensations and allow whatever you experience, even an itch, a feeling of warmth or an ache to enter your awareness.

A phrase I often use is "notice noticing the difference".

Then you open yourself to focus on all your thoughts, sensations, sounds and feelings that enter into your awareness.

There is much research to show that mindfulness may help with stress, pain and chronic health problems like migraines. Mindfulness can be particularly helpful in helping people with their weight loss journey.

When research was done comparing obese women who practiced mindfulness with those in a control group, the mindfulness volunteers reported greater control on their weight loss journey. This helped them with their eating and led to fewer binge eating episodes.

Exercises for Controlled Breathing

1. Sit quietly in a nice space and focus on your breathing.

2. Now take five slow and deep breaths. Notice the air pulling down into your abdomen. Concentrate on your breathing.

3. **Note.** If thoughts do come to mind, as they will do at first, such as "I must collect the shopping on the way home" "Must pick up my prescription" Just let them go in your mind and refocus with the rhythm of your breathing.

4. As you breathe in let your stomach rise and picture yourself inhaling warm, soothing air.

5. As you breathe out, let your stomach fall and now visualize yourself exhaling.

Try this version –

Breathing in, I am calm and careful of what I eat,
Breathing out, I feel in control of my eating.

Walking meditation

This approach uses the rhythm of walking and breathing to stay in the present moment. As you walk, focus on your body. Be aware of your posture. Feel your feet walking along the pavement or around the park as you walk around it. Feel your arms swing. Note your breathing. Keep your mind focused on the present.

Don't allow yourself to get distracted by thoughts or sounds. Don't allow old conversations from the past to resurface as they distract your mind. Walking meditation keeps you mindfully aware of your body. As your awareness grows you'll feel more connected with your body and you'll be less likely to abuse it with unhealthy eating.

Counting – breathing meditation

Focus on breathing and counting your breaths. If you have a few moments try it now. Breathe smoothly in and out. Feel your diaphragm lift and fall as you count up to thirty. Whenever stress builds or the urge to overeat strikes, this exercise can serve as a quick intervention.

Exercise – checking your motive to losing weight

- Close your eyes and let yourself relax. Take a few deep breaths and relax a little deeper each time you exhale.

- Now let your mind drift back to a recent time when you were not hungry but ate something anyway.

- Get in touch with all the details of what is going on. Where are you? Who else is with you? What are you wearing? What's going on?

- Be in the moment before you are about to eat. What are you thinking? What are you feeling? What is going on? CHECK YOUR MOTIVE………….. What do I *really* need in this moment?

- Once you have established this

  (Be honest with yourself and the answer you get, we always know the truth about ourselves)

- Ask "what are other solutions or choices that you can make to fill this need or needs? What else can you do instead of eating that will make you feel better... and more confident in yourself?

- Now go to the time just after eating? What are you thinking?

- Now imagine going to a time when you didn't eat something because you had a made a decision not to this time. Maybe you had a wedding to go to or something of importance and you wanted to look good in your clothes. How did you feel ?

- Now notice the difference between how you felt before and after you eat something you didn't really need.

This exercise will give you an insight to what and why you are eating inappropriately and what you can do to readdress these issues.

This is an another powerful exercise for exploring the reason behind you wanting food in the moment and

Start a positive group.

Group therapy can and has been shown to work very well. With so many meet-up groups now available you are spoilt for choice. The reason they work is because they provide safe and supportive environment where people can share the experiences and discuss their problems around losing weight. Through groups like these, people hear the struggle others face, how they are overcoming them and together can solve issues in ways that maybe they hadn't thought of before.

Maybe you could get a small group together and start your own weight loss discovery group. You don't have to be an experienced group organiser to start your own group. It can work better if it just starts with a few friends and then develops from there. Ask friends, neighbours, work colleagues, mums groups and maybe people from the local gym who can do with extra support without paying a load more money - just don't tell the gym staff.

You will find that when you get like-minded people together you will be surprised by the results you can achieve. You could even do some of the many exercises in this book. Once you get about 6 – 8 people on board then decide where you are going to meet on a regular basis; same place, same time is a good idea, and plan in advance.

It is important to make sure it starts and stops on time as it then looks more professional. Always keep the objective of the meeting in mind otherwise it can easily become just a group of friends having a chat with no positive outcome (in terms of weight loss). Maybe get people to bring in a piece of homework or latest positive research about losing weight; try to not to focus too much on just the latest quick fix.

Perhaps one week you could look and try out new and different exercises, which can be great fun whilst exercising at the same time. It can work well if you get everyone to lead the group in rotation; that way it doesn't get stale and is a good confidence boost for everyone involved.

Even if you don't think of yourself as a group leader or joiner, you may discover unexpected advantages in being in a positive group and you will be also surprised when the weight starts falling off. People will notice and also want to join your successful groupven more so where social media is used to promote new ideas. A group that is confident is always attractive to others.

The positives behind group working can be:-

- Collective problem solving

- Great emotional support

- Laughter and building new friendships

- Encouragement and empathy

- Group workouts

- Support when self-sabotaging creeps in

Getting the best out of your brain.

Left brain or right brain? What is your neurological style? People routinely use both sides of the brain. Much research has shown that there are many differences in the way each side of the brain functions. You need to understand this in order to exploit it during your weight loss and ongoing maintenance programmes.

The brain's right hemisphere controls the muscles on the left side of the body while the left hemisphere controls the muscles on the right side of the body. This side is mainly in charge of spatial abilities, face recognition and processing music. The brain's right side also helps us to comprehend visual imagery and make sense of what we see.

It plays a role in language, particularly in interpreting context and a person's tone.
The general rule of the left side of the brain is that it is dominant in language, processing what you hear and handling most of the duties of speaking. Therefore it is in charge of carrying out logic and exact mathematical computations. When you remember a fact, your left brain pulls it from your memory.

When you are losing weight it's best if you use both sides of the brain. That way you get the best help available. Feed your brain with plenty of facts but use the creativity and imagination side as well.

A good exercise is to write down the most common foods you eat. As you record the information indicate if the food is protein, carbohydrates, calories or fat, including portion size/weight. You will find that you will have them memorized with 2 weeks. Then when you start to cook or go shopping you be able to access the information in your mind.

Then give the creative side of the brain something to do by creating a picture in your mind of you wear that tight fitting dress or those new jeans. Initially, imagine yourself struggling into , imagine the clothes going on really easily and notice how good you feel.

By using both sides of your brain you will find yourself making better food choices for your new healthy lifestyle.

Try this little fun exercise – If you rub the other side of your body, therefore left hand rubs right side of body and right hand rubs left side of body, you will find that you will feel more stimulated as you have used both sides of the brain. Its works really well. Try it.

A little bit of exercise moves you forward.

Starting a weight loss programme and including exercise into your new healthy lifestyle can be hard sometimes and sticking to new routines may at times seem challenging.

There is much research that shows keeping your muscles moving will engage your brain. An example of this would be when you are out running and you're very tired. You notice that your arms will be hanging towards the floor and your legs will feel tired. However, when you start pumping your arms as you run, you find that your legs have more energy and the more you swing your arms the more your legs will work better.

It is also shown that people who keep the positive benefits in their mind show more progress. Remember to keep the following interesting facts in mind when you are next training.

More life in your years = more years in your life.
Physical activity has been shown to slow down the ageing process; therefore, you remain healthier and are more active for longer. If you exercise vigorously and often, which means training a minimum of 30 minutes a day for six days a week, you can actually extend your life and have much more energy.

Maintain a healthy heart. Exercise supplies oxygen to your heart which in turn helps improve the blood flow as well as lowering both your cholesterol levels and blood pressure. If you have high blood pressure then exercise will help a lot.

Exercise protects against cancer. Research shows that moderate exercise such as walking for half an hour most days can significantly reduce the risk of breast cancer. This is a simple and very useful exercise to avoid this terrible disease. Also, active people have been shown to have lower rates of colon and rectal cancer because exercise increases the rate at which waste moves through the digestive system.

Gain stronger bones. Weight training is very good for strength training. If you do weight training two or three times a week it will help and improve bone density and lower vulnerability to bone injury and weakness.

Improve your sleep. Any physical activity reduces the stress chemicals and does reduces the tension levels and because you have exercised you will be more tired and will fall asleep faster, which leads to sleeping longer and when you awaken you will feel much more refreshed.

Enjoy a brighter mood. Studies have shown that taking any form of exercise is just as effective as taking medication in helping to treat mild to moderate depression.

It also increases energy, which in turn reduces anxiety which in turn boosts positive feelings.

Regular exercise will also improve concentration and alertness at any age which, in turn, leads to significant boosts of cognitive functioning in older individuals.

Build greater stamina. With continued exercising, muscles become stronger and in turn function more smoothly, work longer and withstand more strain.

So, as you see from all of the above, there are many benefits to doing some form of exercise. When you start to take control over one aspect of your life, such as exercising, this will have several knock-on effects in other parts of your life.

You will start to feel more confident which, you will be pleased to know will help you lose more weight along your healthy weight loss journey.

You now have a great understanding of how to achieve easy weight loss. This is what you have learned.

1. You have two choices about your weight; Accept it or change it.It is up to you.

2. If you use more positive affirmation techniques, as discussed in this book you will stay on track and achieve great success.

3. You are now much more conscious of what you put into your mouth when you eat.

4. You have a wonderful range of new exercises to do for when you think you have blown it.

5. You are more aware of your comfort foods and you know that after 20 minutes the feeling of hunger will pass; you will be proud you didn't grab some food.

6. You understand what your representational system is now and that of your family and friends.

7. You have a great understanding of EFT (That Tapping Thing) and how you can use it easily to reduce your cravings.

8. You are now taking responsibility and not blaming your genes, family or any other excuse you have used to blame for your weight gain in the past.

9. You are now choosing to take control of the mind set in your head and you choose the correct thoughts that you are in control of.

10. You are always learning more and enjoying this book, as you continue on your successful weight loss journey.

"I wake up every day with the realization that this is it, that there's only one shot at this life and I can either enjoy the ride and live it to its fullest and to my highest potential or I can stay the way I am".

Be inspired, you now have

The Winning Mind Set for Weight Loss

Thank you for completing and reading

The Winning Mind Set For Weight Loss

The Thin Book for Thin People

Be seeing a thinner, more confident you in the near future.

Love and Light Weight

Gary Sellors

Further information and training available:

www.mysilenceisbroken.com – A website and book for helping survivors of Sexual Abuse and Rape

Co-Founder of Healing Connections Magazine, now in its 10th year with a print of over 9000 copies and 3 editions each year.
www.healingconnectionsmagazine.com

Business NLP Training / Coaching / Hypnotherapy / Counselling / CBT / Mindfulness

Past clients include: Harrods, Elstree Film Studios, Heals, House of Fraser, Marks and Spencer, Freedom Communications, John Lewis and many more.

Sports Coaching / Personal Training – Has worked with top UK Athletes who then went on to win British and European gold medals.

Currently part of the Medical Team and Pitch side Medic at Wembley Stadium. Have experience working at the Champions League Final 2013, The Olympics 2012 and the Rugby World Cup Final 2015.

Enjoyed both working with the YMCA Central LondonAs a Positive Health Instructor and with HIV and AIDS groups for just under 2 years.

Currently involved in a new project Positively Mindful – Being Well with HIV Jan 2016

Animal Healing / Animal Behaviour training

Gary Sellors can be contacted on:

- wellbeingconsultant@hotmail.co.uk
- LinkedIn
- www.garyselllors.com

Current books available on Amazon and Kindle plus some local book stores:

- **My Silence is Broken** – A Workbook for Helping Survivors of Sexual Abuse and Rape.

- Future books to look out for:

- Animal healing – Understanding your animals
- Are you Sprouting Out?
- Naturally Feminine – Reshaping your body through the power of your mind
- Colour Your Body
- Improving your eyesight naturally